12/07 donation 12 95

SYMBOLS AND SYMPTOMS

Symbols

AND

Symptoms

In Which Medicine
And Its Relationship to the Humanities
Are Considered

Frank C. Wilson, M.D.

Kenan Professor of Orthopaedics

Instructor in the Humanities,
Undergraduate Honors Curriculum,
University of North Carolina at Chapel Hill

Guild Press of Indiana, Inc.
Indianapolis

GUILD PRESS OF INDIANA, INC.
6000 Sunset Lane
Indianapolis, Indiana 46208

Library of Congress
Catalog Card Number
95-81760

ISBN 1-878208-70-5

Manufactured in the United States of America.

Text design by Sheila Samson
Typefaces: Goudy and Charlemagne

CONTENTS

For the Grandchildren —
Peter, Merrimon, and Ann

FOREWORD

In this set of occasional papers, Frank Wilson shares the mature wisdom of a thoughtful clinician with an extraordinary scope of human and scholarly interest. His perspectives are refreshing, his insights are arresting, and his expressions are both direct and evocative. The collection reflects Dr. Wilson's devotion to the art of exposition of ideas in the context of his probing of the human and scientific dimensions of medical practice and the professional life of the physician.

He treats the interactions of science and the humanities generally and of medicine more specifically. He examines creativity in medicine and the human and social accommodation to medical advances. He discusses values and ethics, teaching, learning and becoming, a bit of biomedical politics and some evolving tensions that are reshaping medical practice.

The thoughtful and eloquent lines of these papers portray Dr. Wilson as he has been known to generations of students, residents, and colleagues: a magnificent teacher.

Stuart Bondurant
Chapel Hill, NC
30 December 1994

PREFACE

These short pieces have been written, usually as addresses, throughout the span of a thirty-year career in academic medicine. Although they come with different labels, each contains thoughts which touch upon the relationship between medicine and the humanities. If they then may be said to have a unifying theme, it is the plea for retention of a humanistic dimension in medicine, whose house is under strong siege by technocracy.

Hoping that the observations would be as valid later as they seemed when they were written, I searched for principles, avoiding the ephemera of "facts" and figures. Stimulated by the writings of Sir William Osler, I had come early to the belief that provision of an ignitional spark was the highest calling of an educator, which led me to reach in each article for an inspirational note.

Although certain issues may lack the sense of urgency that compelled comment in the past, they are included with the hope that reiteration will stir awareness of their continued relevance.

I owe much to many, but would be remiss indeed not to acknowledge my debt to my wife Ann, whose patience and creative insight enabled me to clarify and deepen parts of these essays.

FCW
9 November 1995

THE NEW PHYSICIAN

Mindful of the traditions of the Whitehead Society and of the eminence of previous speakers on this occasion, I stand here with a deep sense of humility and responsibility.

I should like first to congratulate the members of the first-year class on their decision to study medicine. With the changing prestige and autonomy of physicians and the rising cost of medical education, this choice reflects a genuine interest in human welfare and bio-

This essay, delivered as the Whitehead Lecture to students and faculty of the University of North Carolina School of Medicine, September 1, 1967, was published in a slightly different text in *The Bulletin of the University of North Carolina School of Medicine* XV(1):8, 1967.

logical science — qualities that augur well for a successful career in medicine.

My purpose today is not to eulogize our profession. Were you unaware of its worth, you would not be sitting where you are today. Rather, my intent is to consider how we may protect and preserve the ideals upon which medicine is founded — for you and for future generations of physicians.

In recent years, an unprecedented amount of criticism has been directed toward the medical profession, often to the point of overt hostility — and too often with justification. While it may be premature to conclude that medicine is following the course of the Roman Empire, it is clear that currents of social change are eroding its bedrock. The inability of organized medicine to effect needed changes within the profession suggests the difficulties in altering this state by collective action; however, we need not become silent witnesses to our own demise. Our hope lies in the individual physician, for historically it is through singular effort and achievement that medicine has made its most significant advances.

If personal action is to effect meaningful change, it must address the accusations that medicine is failing to meet special needs in both health care and in human relations.

With respect to the quantity and quality of medical care, there *is* ample room for doubt. Even though the doctor-to-patient ratio has increased in recent years, more people are now seeking medical care; and with more physicians engaging in non-patient care activities, such as research and teaching, access to a physician has become more difficult.

As a testimonial to the quality of care, it has been cited that the life span of an average citizen lengthens each year. True, infant mortality has been reduced by better obstetrical care and the control of infectious disease, but the *adult* life span has been extended only slightly since the beginning of the century. In addition, the mounting toll of iatrogenic illness suggests that the first law of the physician — do no harm — has been ignored in the surge of medical science.

Possibly, then, the quality as well as the quantity of medical care can be improved.

The rise of its science — often considered the factual and changeless aspect of medicine — has been attended by a decline in its art; but it is the art, rather than the facts, which is immutable. The need to establish an effective relationship with a patient is critical to the collection of clinical information. Extracting, sifting, weighing, and integrating this knowledge in the context of a person remain the basis of an art which will always be crucial to the care of patients.

Perhaps we may take refuge in research. One has but to consider the medical achievements of vaccine, antibiotic, and organ replacement to feel pride in being part of such a vital profession. Equally visible, but less often seen, is a lack of calculable science in such everyday decisions as when to operate or which drug to use — largely because of a public that demands immediate and dramatic outcomes. As a result, pressing, short-term research goals are often supported, while projects of ultimately greater potential that lack the prospect of an imminent breakthrough go wanting. The art of grantsmanship often overshadows the research itself. You may remember the interview with the mythical Grant Swinger that appeared in *Science* some years ago. He was the director of Breakthrough Institute, a research establishment dedicated exclusively to fulfilling the public demand for scientific breakthroughs. When asked what breakthroughs he had achieved, his answer was that it was difficult to say at this point, but he was pleased to be able to report to the public and the granting agencies a broad variety of imminent break-throughs. And, when queried about the utility of a particular project, the Utilizable Sonic Boom, or USB, Swinger stated that he could not think of any, but they had panelized the problem and given them full responsibility for planning a breakthrough — and the panel had been selected by their standing *ad hoc* committee on panels. While science does not need this type of publicity, it is important to inform the public of the value of scientific inquiry, some of which may have no imme-diate or apparent practical worth.

We must also be careful of the conclusions we draw from research. Observations and even statistics can be misleading, a fact that Mark Twain must have realized when he noted that figures don't lie, but liars figure. The need for caution in the interpretation of research results is illustrated by the story of a scientist who was investigating stimulus and response in the animal laboratory. After stationing a dog in one corner of the room and himself in another he called the animal, whereupon the dog came trotting obediently across the room. Replacing the dog, he tied his two front legs together and called again; this time the dog limped across the room with somewhat more difficulty. The animal was positioned a third time and three legs tied together. The investigator called, and again the animal struggled slowly to his side. In the last phase of the experiment, all of the dog's legs were bound. The scientist called, whistled, and called again, all without effect. The dog lay still on his side in the far corner of the room. Whereupon the investigator recorded the following conclusion: "A dog with all four legs tied together cannot hear."

Thus, even our science might profit from a different perspective.

If we accept the necessity for change, we must decide which changes are needed and how to effect them. We cannot simply wish forth the ideal physician from this or any medical school — regardless of how many times we revise the curriculum. The qualities of change must come from within each physician's personal commitment to excellence — but excellence is a difficult quality to define. What creates it? Why do some people who are innately less well-endowed than others consistently perform in a more superior fashion? Although excellence depends in a measure upon genetic factors, the level at which innate qualities are *expressed* is determined by the commitment, effort, humanism, and integrity that drive them.

Commitment is difficult to define and impossible to measure. If we could quantify desire, predicting success or failure in life would be much easier. The reach of a physician should exceed his grasp, but professional aspirations entail the placement of public ahead of personal welfare. Financial benefit and recognition often follow a dedication to scholarship and truth; the reverse is rarely true. And it is important to realize that scholarship is not restricted to academia. Scholarship is a frame of mind, as indicated by Flexner, who noted that medicine recognized no difference in intellectual attitude between laboratory and clinic, nor between investigator and practitioner; both, he stated, must be acutely conscious of a responsibility to scientific spirit and scientific method.[1] With that approach, the physician will inevitably endeavor to clarify his conceptions and to proceed more systematically in the accumulation of data, the framing of hypotheses, and the evaluation of results. Nor does the pursuit of knowledge stop with graduation. Less and less of what is known and needed to practice medicine will be taught in medical school. The superior physician will remain a student, engaged not in a medical course but in a life course. There will be a tendency to substitute what is euphemistically called wisdom for deteriorating medical knowledge, but there is no substitute for knowing. Nor will it be enough to tether your mind in the field of science. A physician, because he is highly educated, is expected to be well-informed in many areas. To be part of your time, your interests and involvement must span cultural and political as well as scientific issues, so that you may be effective and comfortable in the modern world . . . the true purpose of study.

Central to the concept of commitment is Osler's masterword — "work" — which embraces quality as well as quantity. Excellence will belong not so much to the person who does the most work as to the one doing most of the best work. For work to have direction and purpose, it must possess the quality of method. Aimless effort is like treading water; it may keep you afloat, but it won't take you very far. The virtue of organization will increase in value when, as practicing physicians, you encounter more irregularities of time and obligation. By organizing individual experiences in a meaningful way, you will also develop the capacity for inductive logic that characterizes the successful practitioner.

Nor will everyone work in the same way. Some will be concerned directly with patient care; others will contribute primarily through teaching or research; but all are working toward the same goal — the prevention and cure of illness. Research is the tool whereby an impression is elevated to a level of predictability. Teaching distributes the fruits of research, and practice applies these teachings to patients. Implicit in any area of medical endeavor, however, is the premise that we are here not to draw from but to give back to life. Education is not a one-way street, moving only from faculty to student. It is enhanced by the exchange of ideas. Both the faculty and school should be better for a student's having been there. Unfortunately, there will be a certain amount of seemingly unnecessary and repetitious work, perhaps illustrated by the anecdote of a hospital director who had just received an efficiency report from the president of the board. He finally decided to return the favor to this man who was also president of the board of the local symphony. After listening to several concerts the administrator wrote, "For considerable periods the four oboe players had nothing to do. Their number should be reduced and their work spread more evenly over the whole concert. All twelve first violins were playing identical notes. This seems unnecessary duplication. The staff of this section should be drastically cut. If a large-sound volume is required it could be obtained by electronic amplifier apparatus. There seems too much repetition of some musical passages. Scores should be pruned. No useful purpose is served by repeating on horns a passage already played by strings. It is estimated that if all redundant passages were eliminated the two-hour concert could be reduced to twenty minutes and no intermission needed."

Work brings with it the corollary of thoroughness. Learning in depth is ultimately the most valuable knowledge. First-year students are so caught up in the newness of their adventure that just mastering the language of medicine may seem accomplishment enough; but one must be wary of superficiality. Anchor your knowledge in the sciences of medicine: biology, anatomy, and chemistry; they are the shields against charlatanism.

The third quality of excellence is humanism. Since you will hear much of science during your medical lives, I hope you will not begrudge me a few remarks on the non-science of medicine. There are genes and hormones enough to consume generations of scientific study, but our commitment to the patient is total. The effects of compassion and understanding are more difficult to define than those of morphine or digitalis, but they are often the major determinants of outcome. Science, the basic knowledge of our professional life, must not be substituted for, but added to, the quality of humanism. A student must guard against the replacement of compassion by cynicism as he climbs the ladder of education. An attitude of caring is as important to a physician's success as the possession of medical skills. Remember that we exist for illness, not illness for us — a fact which, with our command of a seller's market, sometimes causes patients to be sacrificed on the altar of personal convenience or medical red tape. The increase in malpractice actions has resulted largely from a lack of basic humanity. The best way to prevent legal intrusion into health care is to maintain warm human relationships with patients, all of whom should be treated with respect and dignity and without prejudgment as to their ability to appreciate or ours to profit from the encounter. Our role is to help; judgements are better left to those in legal or theological professions. People differ in their responses to illness, so we must resist the temptation to classify patients as good or bad.

Coming to terms with the fourth ingredient of excellence — integrity — proved the most challenging part of this essay. It seems clear enough that integrity is the moral essential for excellence, but can it be acquired, and, if so, how? Where human beings live in association, there are problems of conduct, and decisions must be made involving right and wrong. Integrity is soundness of moral principle in making these distinctions. But what makes a thing right or wrong? If one considers this question very long it becomes apparent that there is no single, final, or absolute answer. Custom, law, conscience, religion, and circumstance all play a part in the formulation of moral principles. No one can teach integrity. The quest for it begins with the Socratic dictum, "Know thyself." Before the mind can grasp new truth, its acquired prejudices, ignorance, and presuppositions must be faced and expelled. Honest self-appraisal leads quickly to the realization that one is neither godlike nor omniscient; and awareness of the fine lines between inspiration, perspiration, and pure chance will allow you to rest comfortably under the cloak of humility that characterizes a professional.

Self-knowledge will help you achieve the objectivity and understanding needed to resolve ethical and moral dilemmas that will confront you as practitioners. Your principles will be tested often. There will be times when it is easier to agree or say nothing than to stand and be counted. It may be less difficult to reconcile yourself to accepted but inferior standards of practice than to insist upon their observance; or less troublesome to give a patient what she wants than to explain why she should not have it; or to indulge your ego by joining a patient's criticism of another physician. Although temporarily expedient, such attitudes will wear away the standards upon which medicine is founded. The indications for treatment should be as precise as science will allow. You should refuse any entente with a patient against another physician, stopping short of participation in a protective conspiracy.

Excellence then is an acquired habit, an elixir which when tasted becomes intoxicating and irresistible. It is the best defense against criticism. No debate, political action, or publicity will be as effective as daily excellence in your work as physicians — the services you render without thought of personal gain. I would therefore urge you to develop in yourselves a reluctance to accept anything beneath your best effort, for it is with the tools of excellence that the new physician will be forged. Such a physician, as Stephen Paget noted, may not have reached the top of the tree, but he can still congratulate himself that he is on a branch. "He may be thankful for the natural dignity of his work, its unembarrassed kindness, its insight into life, its hold in science — for these privileges and all that they bring with them will lift him up and up, high over the top of the tree, circle above circle, out of the reach of words."[2]

References

1. Flexner, A. *Medical Education in the United States and Canada.* New York: Report of the Carnegie Foundation for the Advancement of Teaching, 1910.
2. Paget, S. *Confessio Medici.* New York: Macmillan Co., 1908.

Symbols and Symptoms

Although medicine and literature account for much of what is highest and best in my life, to speak or even think convergently, about subjects as manifestly disparate as literature and medicine is a challenging task. Faced, in the sessions of silent thought, with a blank page and a reluctant pencil, I wondered if there was anything I might say about the context of humanity in which science serves medicine that had not been more profoundly and eloquently expressed by C. P. Snow, Peter Medawar, and perhaps a half-dozen others.

This essay was published in a slightly different text in *Perspectives in Biology and Medicine* 32(3):449–54, 1989.

A spark was struck by rereading a 1967 address to the medical students, in which I had cautioned them not to let their humanism be cancelled by a more rapidly evolving science — apprehension then, overarching reality today. True, the ballpark has changed and the rules are different now, but the "facts" upon which we base decisions have always been fleeting. Lasting solutions are elusive, but the absence of any final answer to the decline of humanism in science should not prevent a search for higher ground — nor from acknowledging that our preoccupation with technology has all but routed humanistic and philanthropic concerns; and, since each methodological advance must be managed by an even more sophisticated technology, the imbalance is likely to increase. So captivated are we by the prospect of the next technical breakthrough that too little thought is given to the role of the last one. As a result of what can be done, health care expectations have become unrealistically inflated; in fact, we have so titillated the public with this display of methodological muscle that failure to cure has become tantamount to breaking the law. But complete health care for every American is no longer an option. Given rising economic and ecologic limitations, the choice is no longer whether, but how medical care will be rationed. What then can be done to equip its providers with the wisdom and judgement they will need to make these complex ethical decisions?

Knowledge alone is insufficient. The skill of a physician relates to his ability to give a specific fact appropriate dimension and location within the context of an entire person; but the application of scientific data to the human condition requires greater educational diversity than is provided in conventional curricula. Undergraduates simply don't maintain their horizontal dimension long enough. Certainly baccalaureate education should include the fundaments for a career in science, but elective courses, potentially valuable for achieving educational diversity, are too often chosen simply to fatten grade point averages or to ease the transition to medical school. I have no quarrel with — would, in fact, support strongly — those who seek in science a rigorous and disciplined education; but rigor and discipline are hallmarks of scholarship in other subjects as well. The answers in nonscientific fields may be less precise or conclusive, but the search for truth is no less rigorous or demanding. Medicine itself is an inexact science. Normal is never a point but a range, and most patients have problems for which there are no single, perfect answers.

Of particular value are courses that stress concepts and principles, logic and analysis. History and poetry are also relevant, not so much to master dates or couplets as to obtain a sense of history and poetry. Nor should a general education omit courses in self-expression, such as public speaking and expository writing. Basic reading and writing skills have been impoverished by the substitution of pictures for words — an unfortunate necessity for the twenty-seven million Americans who are functionally illiterate.

My first awareness of the connection between medicine and literature occurred when I was advised as a third year medical student to read the "literature" on a particular topic. Until that time, my associations with the word "literature" involved the spires of Oxford and the high poetry of Dante. Certainly the word didn't have medical connotations, although as I became better acquainted with such works as *The Anatomy of Melancholy*, I realized that the phrase "medical literature" was neither an oxymoron nor a crime against nature. Nevertheless, I'm still a little uneasy about public meetings of the two, feeling, somewhat like Chekhov, that my lawful wife is medicine and literature my mistress, and it is just as well to keep the two apart in polite society.

The differences are obvious: literature is subjective and fanciful — a matter of taste; medicine is objective and rational — a matter of fact. In medicine, ideas must be verified before they can be accepted. Literature is more comfortable with ideas that may never be proven, realizing that the meaning of life is not found in DNA sequences.

Similarities are less conspicuous, but both literature and medicine seek a fundamental understanding of humanity. There is no profession, perhaps other than the ministry, which deals more with mankind in moments of trouble, birth, illness, and death than medicine. Therefore, understanding humanity is not only relevant, but critical; and whatever part of that understanding is learned must be derived from personal and vicarious experience. Since personal contact with illness and bereavement is limited, we rely on the descriptions of others for further insight into the human condition. Through the sadness and joy, tragedy and triumph of its characters, literature provides such diverse and humanizing moments. Indeed, the best literature is the most varied and far-ranging. Those authors with only one story to tell (although they may tell it many times) are comparable to physicians fixed in a highly specialized technology who, lacking flexibility, make patients fit procedures rather than tailoring procedures to the needs of patients.

Of course most of us don't read for its humanizing value. We read for the enchantment and the stories, to escape boredom or some unpleasantness in life. "Once upon a time" are among the most evocative and best-remembered words of childhood and still convey for many of us a sense of magical and faraway adventure.

Another similarity is that both medicine and literature tell a story. The physician's history is a tale of disorder, disease, and death; from the writer's view, these occurrences are woven into the tapestry of everyday life. It may not be fortuitous that the decline in the art of medical history-taking has coincided with a diminishing interest in good literature.

Authors and physicians appear to use different tools: authors employ symbols, physicians rely on symptoms; but the term "symbol," as first used by the Greeks, referred to original wholeness, later broken, then forever sought. Symptoms, too, reflect an incompleteness for which we seek relief. Both may be as obvious as the representation of a country by its flag; at other times, however, both symbols and symptoms have been passed through filters of emotion, attitude, life-style, stress, and guilt. Placing these symbols and symptoms in the context of their full meaning may require some detective work, but therein lie the real challenges of medical diagnosis and literary comprehension. Contact with subconscious meanings in literature makes us more aware of their existence in patients. In this sense, literature enlarges our sensitivities and our imagination; it may not help us listen, but it enables us to hear better.

The creative process is also similar for writers and scientists, although creation in scientific fields must deal with a larger canon of technology and fact between creative insight and its expression. Great writers, like great physicians, reach fundamental truth through conscious and unconscious distillation of many separate observations. The power of these truths depends upon the clarity and wholeness of the observations. Unfortunately, most of us use only part of our sensory equipment, but our powers of perception may be increased by using all our senses. Literature reaches the senses through the mind and thus has the broadest application to the human condition; but music and art also have benefit: music makes us aware of variations in sound, cadence, and rhythm, and art heightens our consciousness of form and color. Thus, literature, music, and art add to science by giving greater depth and force to the physician's observations. With the intensified sensibilities resulting from full use of our faculties, the faces of disease literally jump out of a crowd. So prepared, one may identify many abnormalities of form and function with no more equipment than a park bench.

I am sometimes asked why I teach a course in literature. What is meant is why is a surgeon doing something for which he is certainly unprepared and probably unsuited. Hoping to avoid an immediate and full disclosure of

my incompetence, I have replied — as enig-
matically as possible — that it gives me the
opportunity to fulfill a socially acceptable
fantasy. Some nod uneasily, murmur something
like, "Oh, I see," and move on. Others, determined to get to the bottom of this in-
congruous incongruity, follow with, "But why
Thomas Wolfe?" "Why not?" seems to be a
rather unsatisfying response, so I go on, my
defense having become more elaborate with
time. Somebody should be teaching him, I
suggest, since by his ability to evoke through
language the American dream, he is one of
our most important writers. For any who still
are listening, I point out that the English
language is in a state of decline, that increasing exposure to preformed images is remov-
ing the stimulus and opportunity for exercise
of our own imaginations, and this course is
my vote for the written word over its picto-
rial representation.

Physicians must understand that medicine is not limited to the repair of mechanical parts; that methodological approaches are like sex manuals: the larger pleasure may be lost in preoccupation with technique. The biological aspects of medicine must be applied in the context of understanding and humanity. The fact that one dies of his entire life, not just of his disease, doesn't mean that literature should be substituted for science in medicine; rather, their effect should be additive, so that literature gives increased meaning to the physician's findings. Literature is a window on life that promotes understanding, enhances communication, and keeps tradition and memory alive. It instructs our science by providing a sense of wholeness, thus balancing the forces of specialization, which tend to focus on parts rather than people. Once a patient is seen or remembered as an organ or an x-ray, at that very moment he ceases being an individual.

Good literature goes even further; it has the power to show rather than simply tell us what happened. Flaubert's portrayal in *Madame Bovary* of a country surgeon's disastrous attempts to correct a clubfoot illustrates more vividly than any lecture the critical importance of knowledge and skill to the art of healing:

> The taliped was twisting about in dreadful convulsions; the apparatus in which his foot was encased was hitting the wall hard enough to smash it.
>
> Taking many precautions so as not to disturb the position of the limb, they pulled off the box. A hideous sight was revealed. The foot was swollen to an unrecognizable shape, the skin seemed about to burst open. . . . But hardly had the swelling subsided when the two scientists decided it was time to put the foot back in the apparatus. They even tightened it to obtain quicker results. Finally, three days later, when Hippolyte could not endure it any longer, they removed the mechanism once more. They were greatly surprised at the result which greeted them. A livid tumescence

was spread all over the leg, dotted with blisters oozing a dark liquid.[1]

Certainly there is no textbook description that portrays the ugliness, beauty, and power of death more graphically than Thomas Wolfe's moving recollections of the deaths of his brother and father. Describing the untimely death of Ben from pneumonia, Wolfe wrote,

The rattling in the wasted body, which seemed for hours to have given over to death all of life that is worth saving, had now ceased. The body appeared to grow rigid before them. Slowly, after a moment, Eliza withdrew her hands. But suddenly, marvellously, as if his resurrection and rebirth had come upon him, Ben drew upon the air in a long and powerful respiration; his gray eyes opened. Filled with a terrible vision of all life in the one moment, he seemed to rise forward bodilessly from his pillows without support — a flame, a light, a glory — joined at length in death to the dark spirit who had brooded upon each footstep of his lonely adventure on earth; and, casting the fierce sword of his glance with utter and final comprehension upon the room haunted with its gray pageantry of cheap loves and dull consciences and on all those uncertain mummers of waste and confusion fading now from the bright window of his eyes, he passed instantly, scornful and unafraid, as he had lived, into the shades of death.[2]

And Wolfe's father finds in death the path to a creative life:

Gant was aware that some one had entered the house, was coming towards him through the hall, would soon be with him. Turning his head towards the door he was conscious of something approaching with the speed of light, the instancy of thought, and at that moment he was filled with a sense of inexpressible joy, a feeling of triumph and security he had never known. Something immensely bright and beautiful was converging in a flare of light, and at that instant, the whole room blurred around him, his sight was fixed upon that focal image in the door, and suddenly the child was standing there and looking towards him. . . .

For now the child — or someone in the house — was speaking, calling to him; he heard great footsteps, soft but thunderous, imminent, yet immensely far, a voice well-known, never heard before. He called to it, and then it seemed to answer him; he called to it with faith and joy to give him rescue, strength, and life, and it answered him and told him that all the error, old age, pain and grief of life was nothing but an evil dream; that he who had been lost was found again, that his youth would be restored to him and that he would never die, and that he would find again the path he had not taken long ago in a dark wood.

And the child still smiled at him from the dark door; the great steps, soft and powerful, came ever closer, and as the instant imminent approach of that last meeting came intolerably near, he cried out through the lake of jetting blood, "Here, Father, here!" and heard a strong voice answer him, "My son!"[3]

How, why, or even if these deaths affect you is a reflection of something in you: a brother who died, an unfulfilled life, or simply not having a brother or knowing one's father. Death and disease exist in the context of people. They are woven into the life, emotions, and thoughts of human beings — and those around them (a context, incidentally, that was largely lost when doctors stopped making house calls). For the reason that each patient is an individual, the response to his disease is unique and requires more than knowledge of the disorder itself for its complete understanding. Similarly varied are the effects of illness and death on family and friends. Some are driven apart by a dying relative; others are drawn together in the final communion of death. Thus, the vicarious experiences of literature enable the physician to infuse objective thought and action with greater empathy for the impact of disease or death, not just upon organs or patients, but also upon the lives of those around them. We may never know the full meaning of existence, nor of the life we try so hard to prolong, but we must keep searching for it all along the way — with all the sense and sensitivity we can command.

References

1. Flaubert, G. *Madame Bovary*. M Marmur (trans-ed). New York: Penguin Books Inc., 1964. 177.
2. Wolfe, Thomas. *Look Homeward, Angel*. New York: Charles Scribner's Sons, 1929. 465.
3. Wolfe, Thomas. *Of Time and the River*. New York: Charles Scribner's Sons, 1935. 267–68.

LITTERAE, SCIENTIA, ET HUMANITAS

It is difficult to assemble the dilemmas of modern medicine under one title; in fact, my search for a title brought to mind the account — perhaps apocryphal — of a young writer who approached Somerset Maugham for help in finding a title for a story he had written. "Does your story have any drums?" asked Maugham. "No," said the youth. "Any bugles?" and the author again admitted that it didn't. "Well, then it's easy," said Maugham. "Call it *No Drums, No Bugles*." While this essay suffers the same omissions, I realized as I began to order my thoughts that they fell comfortably

This essay was published in a slightly different text in *Clinical Orthopaedics and Related Research* 150:308–11, 1980.

under the headings of letters, science, and humanism.

Letters refers to the ability to speak and write precisely and clearly; *Science* speaks not only to mastery of known material but also to the development of new knowledge by application of the scientific method; *Humanism* refers to those basic values and qualities of the human spirit that make a physician sensitive to the feeling of his patients and to the social consequences of his actions.

Each of these facets of the complete physician is threatened by changes in the modern world: the humanities are compressed by exploding technology; basic science is diminished by curricular emphasis on behavioral science and by federal disenchantment with fundamental research; and many human values have been lost along the road to pot and the quick fix.

If medicine is to have a meaningful voice

in shaping its destiny, its spokesmen must be able to speak and write with clarity, logic, and perception, because it is they who must present the case for medicine — for preserving what is good and changing what is bad. Unfortunately, those who can articulate clearly with tongue or pen are becoming harder to find because it is no longer necessary to read or write well to function adequately in society. Given that one can now get along adequately without it, the surprise is perhaps that people read as much as they do. And there is little assurance that reading and writing skills will receive increased attention by future educators. One can hardly expect teachers who are themselves products of the television era to lead the counterrevolution.

But television has not been the only influence in the rout of the humanities. They are also retreating from the onslaught of the social sciences, which are said to be more relevant

— as though practicality were the only goal in life. One should search the sky as well as his own footprints for direction. Abstractions may not put a car in every garage or indoor plumbing in every home, but it is abstract thought, the family of ideas, that separates a scholarly profession from a trade union. A primary distinction between a professional and an artisan lies in the breadth of the professional's education — as opposed to the pure vocational training of the craftsman.

Surgery is particularly susceptible to becoming a guild. Its technology has become so complex that surgeons are perforce less involved with other critical elements of patient care. An intellect that grasps principles will find its own methods, but a mind tethered in technology will never develop the perspective needed for sapient judgement.

No single group of subjects assures a balanced education, but philosophy, literature, history, and writing should be included on any list. Courses in expository writing are valuable, not to produce literary masterpieces but to improve written accuracy, clarity, and brevity, so that we may avoid the "obligatory obfuscation" of medical literature. A writer must suppose that his reader is in trouble most of the time — like a man sinking in a swamp — and it is the writer's duty to drain off as much of the water as possible. The cumbersome, pedantic, stereotyped phrasing seen in most medical writing is sometimes believed to indicate a sense of style. It does not. Style is more a reflection of the personality and feelings of the author than it is tricks of grammar or phraseology.

The second pillar of medicine, science, involves the transmission of known material, or teaching, and the development of new knowledge, or research.

Mastery of the basic sciences of medicine

has, since the time of Flexner,[1] enjoyed the status of a "given" in medical education. This core, however, has been eroded by other curricular pressures, to the detriment of medical science. To reestablish the importance of basic science, lay people need to understand more about it — how discoveries are made; how one finding may lead to another, and why, even if there is no obvious or direct benefit, understanding the nature of things around us is a worthwhile goal in itself. We have courses in music and art appreciation — why not science appreciation?

In medical school, our primary obligation is to fundamental knowledge and to the acquisition of attitudes and habits that will assure continued professional development during a lifetime of practice. In spite of the increasing orientation of students toward techniques, the "how to's" of procedures must never be allowed to replace the "why's" of anatomy, physiology, and biochemistry. Without fundamental knowledge, a physician is little more than a technician, for whom a doctoral degree is probably unnecessary.

The problems in graduate education are more numerous and less distinct, and, for these reasons, harder to cope with. In addition to the lack of specific educational goals, there are philosophical dichotomies that defy solution by even the most balanced intellect. Consider the lines of tension between medical and paramedical roles, medical schools and teaching hospitals, the need to develop operative skills and the commitment to patient safety, and between the quality and the cost of medical care.

There are even problems with teachers — not them, but us. We are overtraveled and overcommitted, and, as a result, undercommitteed to bedside teaching and individual clinical practice.

Our loss of dedication to bedside teaching and personalized practice is a product, in part, of the full-time system, an approach promulgated by Flexner in the early part of the century.[1] Flexner was, by all accounts, a superb teacher. He knew his subjects and his students well; he built upon their strengths and challenged them with discipline and single-minded dedication to learning, but he did not achieve his greatness as a teacher by his advocacy of the full-time system. His hope that professors, freed from the demands of private practice, would devote more time to teaching and research was appropriate for his time and was realized. It may be that, as Osler predicted, the pendulum has swung too far. The practice of medicine cannot be taught from the laboratory or even from the classroom. It must be taught at the bedside, in the operating room, and in the clinic. In devoting so much thought to the ingredients of education — to courses and curricula — we sometimes forget that attitude, not content or technique, is the fuel of learning. The basic elements are a faculty who loves to teach and students who want, more than anything else, to learn. Some structure is desirable, but too much direction produces a grooved and complacent student — one whose life, as MacNab has said, is not on a bus but a trolley.

The characteristics of a great teacher are difficult to define. They seem to have little in common except enthusiasm and mastery of subject. Some teach with a bludgeon, some with a scalpel, and some just change their neckties every day. Toughness should perhaps be included among the shared traits, especially in an era when commitment to the quality of the educational offering has already given way to student pressures for reduced educational rigor. A teacher should never be callous or rude, but students should be treated like everyone else — the way they deserve to be treated.

During the period of federal munificence that produced the scientific era of medicine, the medical center gradually became more an institute for research than a focus for learning. Provision of medical care was subsumed by the housestaff, while the practice skills and acumen of the faculty declined. The reversibility of this clinical atrophy has been tested by the decline in research support; however, even if the teaching physician can avoid the assorted administrative snares on his way back to the wards, it is not clear that the strict full-time system can provide the rewards necessary to keep him there. Taking care of the sick requires an enormous amount of time, energy, and emotional commitment. If academic medical centers are to survive in the service marketplace, the financial *modus operandi* must be organized along the lines of multidisciplinary clinics, with a physician incentive system which recognizes patient care activities.

The other aspect of science is the creation of new knowledge. The previous remarks about education and its relation to clinical practice should not be interpreted as denigrating research. Research is essential for the evolution of medical practice and should be fostered early in the educational process. It is an important aspect of medical education because it trains the mind to function both creatively and critically, a necessity in the practice of every physician. The scientific method is perhaps the most powerful tool of the intellect. There is very little difference between physicians — whether researchers or clinicians — who are committed to excellence. Both groups will employ the scientific method: they will frame hypotheses, collect data, and evaluate their results critically. Research not only provides training in the scientific method, but it also lessens the anxiety students have about research. The lack of enthusiasm for investigation during the graduate years often reflects only ignorance of research methodology. However, research need not emanate from a laboratory; many discoveries of fundamental importance have been made, and must continue to be made, in the clinical arena. The important ingredients are critical thinking and recognition of the difference between validated and unvalidated hypotheses.

The last and least tangible part of this address deals with humanism — the conscience, morality, sensitivity, compassion, and commitment of an individual that, more than knowledge or technique, determine what a physician *does*. And it is performance, not competence or ability, that should concern us. In a sense, the complete physician may be likened to an iceberg with its tip of knowledge and skill that can be easily seen and measured. Attitudinal qualities are less visible, but like the submerged portion of the iceberg, are the major determinants of size and shape.

Many basic human values are moving into confrontation with contemporary medicine. Gender, once a given, is now an option. Genetically determined traits are subject to control. The prolongation of life, seemingly a triumph, poses serious ecologic dilemmas. The precepts and norms of biology and mortality are becoming less clear, forcing us to create our own value systems. We must now make decisions where before there was no choice. Considering the magnitude of these judgements, a sense of anxiety and uncertainty is inescapable. It is hard to change from the belief that an abortionist is a criminal to a system that esteems him as a hero. But like it or not, physicians will be asked to defend the social consequences of their actions as well as their effect on individual patients. The choice is whether to make these decisions casually or thoughtfully. The development of a personal philosophy of medicine will require more intense internal analysis than most of us have been accustomed to. New students, not having to fight through so many preconceived notions, may have less trouble. Even so, we should examine our role as teachers in promoting the development of a personal ethic and humanity among students. Can one teach these qualities? Certainly not by lecture alone. Honesty, humility, and compassion are best taught by precept and example, when a student is able to witness these qualities during the interaction between patient and physician. If a student observes his mentors treating patients only as objects of science or as instruments to verify a theory, that student will emulate this pattern in his own practice. In a sense, the physician is like the conductor of a symphony who fuses the knowledge and technology of an orchestra with his own spirit, feeling, and values.

These then are the qualifications for the complete physician: breadth of education, scientific competence, and inner sensitivity. The ingredients must be mixed, seasoned, and simmered in the kettle of practice. Thus, prepared, the physician who emerges can be expected to achieve the goal of excellence in his professional life.

References

1. Flexner, A. *Medical education in the United States and Canada.* New York: Report of the Carnegie Foundation for the Advancement of Teaching, 1910.

CREATIVITY IN MEDICINE

The importance of creativity in any field is plain. It is also clear that much of the responsibility for creating new medical knowledge rests with faculties of medicine, who, in addition to their own contributions, must play a major role in nurturing the creative potential of future physicians. Therefore, in approaching the subject of creativity in medicine, my perspective is that of a concerned faculty member. I hope to justify the relevance of my remarks on four premises:

This essay was published in a slightly different text in *Perspectives in Biology and Medicine* 29 (2):310–15, 1986, under the title "Creativity in Medicine — A Faculty Perspective."

first, the importance of creation in supplying a natural order for man-made disarray; second, that some capacity for creation exists in everyone (whether the *product* of that creativity affects one or many lives is determined by individual genotype, and the extent to which this genetic uniqueness is altered by outside influences); third, that the educational process contains many impediments to creative expression, some of which are correctable; and, fourth, that the enhancement of creative potential is not only possible but a necessary and proper function of a medical educator.

Creativity has been variously interpreted. My use of the word is in the sense of bringing something new into existence by recognizing a relationship between previously unassociated elements. Implicit in this definition are a product and the notion that human creation results not *ex nihilo* but from the use of existing material in unusual ways.

Creativity may be further described by the traits most often associated with it. Creative individuals are more likely to be curious, sensitive, and persistent and to possess the capacity for intense concentration, a high tolerance for ambiguity, and the faculty for divergent thought. Divergent thinking, which enables one to perceive similarities among previously dissimilar elements, is more critical to the creative process than convergent thought, which depends on recall and application of learned material. An aptitude for convergent thinking and high intelligence are frequently associated; however, above an IQ of a hundred and twenty, intelligence has not been shown to be related to creativity.[1]

Further shape may be given to the concept of creativity by understanding what it is not. For example, the simple enumeration of facts increases our knowledge but produces no remarkable insight or novel design. Patience, precision, and even daring are required to count the number of quills on a porcupine, but nothing new has resulted.

Nor is the simple act of discovery creation. Finding an apple that has fallen from a tree is not creative; but by connecting the forces that caused the apple to fall with those "requisite to keep the moon in its orb," Newton made an inductive leap that is the essence of creativity.[2]

Finally, it is important to distinguish creation from interpretation. While the renowned actor may receive more acclaim than the author of a play, it is the latter who created the piece in which the actor performs — however skillfully.

Creativity has both vertical and horizontal dimensions. The vertical plane encompasses the levels of creativity, ranging from simple expressive originality to complex forms of abstraction. Expressive creativity may be verbal or physical, a clever phrase or a unique dance movement, with the product assuming only minor importance. Abstraction leads to a new principle or law of nature, with the product having major significance. Between the expressive and abstract levels is innovation, wherein the application of known principles, technology, or information provides a better way of doing something, of controlling the world around us.

The horizontal dimension embraces the types of creativity. Although the urge to create is largely independent of professional training, creation in artistic fields differs from that in science by having a smaller canon of technology and fact between the creative spark and its expression. Thus, artistic creation is less influenced by conscious thought than scientific discovery, although the flash of illumination that springs from unconscious thought occurs in both. The

"Eureka!" of Archimedes as he stepped into the bathtub resulted from a sudden association similar to the spontaneous apposition of thought and feeling that produced a Wordsworthian ode. Such inductive leaps, however, being intuitive, are sometimes wrong. In science, the generalizations that result must be followed by hypothesis and experiment — the scientific method — which entail conscious connections, logic, and analytical thought.

It is, then, a blend of inspiration and analysis that has produced the peaks of creative achievement in medicine. And although we may be justly proud of past accomplishments, a steady decline of physician-investigators clouds the future of scientific discovery. That the causes for this decline are not based on genetic incompetence is suggested by the report of Gough, whose study showed that medical students had greater creative potential than architects, engineers, mathematicians, or research scientists.[3] Thus, the influences must be external, and those (we, not they) with the best opportunity to extract the innovation from this potential must accept the responsibility for any failure to do so.

Our influence probably starts much earlier than we realize, perhaps the first time we offer a child an ice cream cone for building a sand castle — and by this careless introduction to the marketplace encourage him to work for external rewards rather than the inner pleasure of doing.

Further discouragement occurs in elementary school, where to be different is to be disorderly or disruptive. The need for structure and discipline encourages convergent rather than divergent behavior. Exceptional sensitivity and skill are required of a teacher to preserve classroom order and simultaneously allow creative minds to expand. The student who, when asked to draw a house, depicts the inside rather than the expected outside should be praised, not criticized, for this deviation from the ordinary.

Another characteristic of those bent toward medicine, whether innate or acquired, is an hypertrophied work ethic. Although the essentiality and value of hard work are undeniable, continually focusing on the next course or the next patient reduces the time for free association and creative thought. This preoccupation with task completion — on becoming rather than being — narrows perspectives; other dimensions disappear. An initially diverse group of medical students, homogenized by customary forms of dress, language, and practice, come to look, sound, and act alike.

Embryological research has shown that organisms act on their environment before reacting to it — so perhaps the inclination to work is congenital.[4] But creativity, like many natural phenomena, is a cyclic process in which effort and relaxation, work and play, are balanced. Unfortunately, our culture equates relaxation with idleness, perceiving it more as a reward for work than its necessary diastole. Virtue and achievement are measured by the length of time that effort can be sustained; however, such unrelieved activity has an undesirable side effect: it reduces the time for wonder, for understanding the world around us, and for seeing the unusual in the ordinary.

Even our nonprofessional pastimes tend toward competitive and self-improvement modes. What we are not very good at is loafing, doing nothing. Actually, doing nothing requires self-assurance and intelligence of a high order. Tell your friends that you are doing nothing, and they won't believe you. Their eyes will narrow suspiciously, and they will say things like "Aw, c'mon, what are you really doin'?" They will believe anything but nothing. They will accept you as a cocaine addict or a sex offender — but doing nothing? Never! Our Judeo-Christian training tells us that we are supposed to be producing something, making things add up, getting ahead. But doing nothing is not easy; it takes practice. Of course, the more you do it, the easier it gets; and, after a while, even the guilt subsides.

It would be comforting to believe that individuality is less constrained by the medical phase of education, but such a hope is more romance than reality. Even the process by which medical students are selected favors the convergent stereotype; an amiable personality, conservative dress, and a dignified demeanor curry favor with admissions committees. But these are not traits usually found in creative individuals. Even were we willing to accept scores on standardized tests, there are no indices for creativity in the Medical College Admission Tests.

Nor do we do much better during the educational experience. The traditional authoritarianism of medicine, an enormous amount of factual material, and the pervasive multiple-choice test encourage a black-or-white, yes-or-no type of thought that allows little room for ambiguity. No one relishes intellectual purgatory, but students need to realize that some questions have many answers; others none. They must understand that uncertainty and anxiety are inevitable — and therefore acceptable — emotions. Perhaps, as Cohen suggested, we should have "uncertainty rounds" which deal only with patients whose problems have no single or best answer.[5]

Finally the student escapes the stultifying effect of classroom and mentor. What then? Some enter practice, where stereotypical behavior is fostered by societal expectations and peer pressure. Others become faculty members, where their creative lives become emasculated by bureaucratic detail, Sisyphean labors, and the quest for increasingly elusive grant support. Thus, to be successful in today's world, the medical scientist must be not only *Homo sapiens* (man the thinker) but also *Homo laboris* (man the worker) — and *Homo "miserium"* (man the miser). Of course, if "buzzing, blooming confusion" is, as James suggested, a condition of creativity, the university milieu is certainly more asset than impediment.[6]

As I said at the beginning, some of these lesions are remediable, and the appropriate therapists are the medical faculty. The first step is to identify those who are unusually imaginative, since the innovative applicant is not set apart by present methods of selection. Psychometric indices of creativity should be incorporated into college and medical school admission tests. The critical incident technique might also be used to identify students possessing those traits most highly correlated with creative behaviors.

We must also insist on greater undergraduate diversity, so that students can maintain their horizontal dimension as long as possible. Verticality will come shortly enough. Special emphasis should be given to courses that stress concepts and principles, logic and analysis, and metaphorical activity. Both analytical and metaphorical processes are needed by the creative scientist. Analysis divides, categorizes, and emphasizes differences; metaphor relates, unites, and stresses similarities. Philosophy is vital because it encourages analysis and discipline, and above all, a search for truth. And, lest we forget, a course in expository writing, so that the rest of us will not have to slog through the swamp of medical writing.

Having ensured the native inventiveness and intellectual breadth of the students, it should be only a matter of time until we get out of the box more than we put in. Perhaps the most important thing now is not to cancel out a student's individuality by insisting that he adopt a particular system of thought, action, or values. If you feel an uncontrollable urge to do something, think about how to make room in your life for creative students. Fanning the spark requires little beyond an attitudinal adjustment and minor modifications in the warp and woof of the curricular cloth: basic and clinical science should be tightly interwoven, passive interlaced with active learning experiences, and periods of intense memorization blended with time to assimilate and apply. Whether the fabric that results is attractive and enticing or dull and uninteresting will depend on the attitudinal coloring, on how much we reflect enjoyment of what we are doing rather than in its rewards.

Once the spark is lit, fuel can be provided by a period of research, free from clinical responsibilities. But a neophyte investigator should not be simply taken off the wards and told to go and "do some research." Young investigators need guidance, financial support, technical help, and access to equipment if they are to have a positive and productive experience in the laboratory. Direction is particularly critical in framing the questions for study and in planning the experiments to test hypotheses generated by these questions. Considerable experience and knowledge of the field are necessary to "set in" the other pieces in the puzzle that determine the size and shape of those being sought.

Although a positive experience is perhaps more likely if the interests and enthusiasms of the investigator are captured in the project, it does not matter greatly whether the research is in basic or applied science as long as the problems are addressed through rigorous application of the scientific method. Even if the research period produces no "Eureka!" experiences and the Nobel Prize goes to another, the enhanced appreciation of scientific methodology and the ability to examine with a more critical eye are justifiable outcomes.

It is felt by some that clinical and research training are not miscible, that they require different attributes and skills; however, research and practice are more akin than antithetical; for both, the scientific method is a conduit to the highest goal of professionalism — the creation of new knowledge. Man cannot create from nothingness, which must be left to a higher being; but may he not pray — as in the majestic passage from *The Divine Comedy* beginning "O highest light" — for the power to leave one spark of God's glory to "the race to come?" So endowed with the divine spark of creation, he may "the universe unfold; all properties of substance and of accident behold."[7]

References

1. Vernon, P. E. *Creativity*. Baltimore: Penguin, 1970.
2. Newton, Sir Isaac. *Encyclopaedia Britannica*, W. Yust, ed. Chicago, 1956.
3. Gough, H. G. "What happens to creative medical students?" *Journal of Medical Education*. 51 (1976): 461–67.
4. Martin, A. R.: "Cultural impairment of our inner resources: An empirical study." *American Journal of Psychoanalysis*. 32 (1972): 27–46.
5. Cohen, M. L. "Uncertainty rounds." JAMA 250 (1983): 1689.
6. Gowan, J. C., G. D. Demos, and E. P. Torrance. *Creativity: Its Educational Implications*. New York: Wiley, 1967.
7. Dante. *The Divine Comedy*. Garden City, New York: Doubleday, 1947.

MEDICAL CURRICULA

PROBLEMS AND PRESCRIPTIONS

W hen asked to speak on the subject of curricula, my acceptance followed the anatomical pathway of a knee reflex, completely bypassing my cerebrum. Even when advised that my comments should be limited to the graduate arena, I saw no cause for panic. After all, curriculum is an overarching theme of the educator's life, and graduate education is, for many of us, the keystone of this arch, so talking about curriculum development seemed an appropriate and reasonable undertaking. However, the longer I stared at the words "Medical

Address to International Symposium of Academic Orthopaedic Manpower, Hershey, Pennsylvania, November 30, 1983.

Curricula," which I had written neatly at the top of the page as I began preparing these remarks, the more convinced I became that the curriculum tiger is particularly carnivorous, sharp of tooth, many-striped — and probably untamable.

I do not want to extend the analogy to suggest that curriculum is a beast to be controlled with whip and chair, but perhaps it does warrant our attention and respect.

Someone has said there are three qualities that every man believes himself to possess, and which, if challenged, will provoke a belligerent response: his ability to drive an automobile, his seductive powers, and his ability to teach. Motor vehicle accident statistics and the data of Masters and Johnson suggest the mythical nature of the first two, and one has only to read the comments made by students in response to our educational efforts to wonder if they, too, are not suspect.

However, the ratings of our educational offerings are less a product of curriculum design than of the ability, enthusiasm, and commitment of the teacher. One of the things curriculum is *not* is a substitute for personal involvement in the educational process. Nor does it provide a destination for the educational experience. Curriculum is only an instrument for getting there, and like any instrument, it requires a guiding hand — the educational goals — to place it where it can exert its greatest leverage. So the objectives of the program must be established first.

It is probably not too far off the mark to suggest that the primary goal of medical education is to produce physicians who blend science with humanism like warp and woof in the practice of medicine. Application of the scientific method is as important in practice as in research because it provides the means by which information may be collected, analyzed, and applied. Stated another way, the scientific method is the discipline that a mind possesses, which is more valuable, especially for educational growth, than any particular furnishings it has.

Unfortunately, the attitudinal and humanistic qualities that are most important for the practice of medicine have not been clearly defined, perhaps because they differ — at least in degree — among the various special fields of medicine. Even if they could be enumerated, how, or whether, they can be taught is a contested issue.

With this rather philosophical underpinning, perhaps we can define some of the specific ills that beset medical curricula and offer prescriptions for their management.

Since it is impossible to deal comprehensively with graduate education without considering the base upon which it stands, we should commence with the deficiencies in undergraduate education that impede development of the skills and attitudes necessary for *continued* learning and problem solving.

First is the failure to use well-known principles of adult learning in the education of medical students, especially during the first two years: we do not show them why they need to know; they are not actively involved in the learning process; and feedback, when it occurs, is often late and impersonal.

Second, there is inadequate diversity throughout the educational continuum, especially in the collegiate years, which produces physicians with a long vertical but a short horizontal dimension.

Third, the lack of linkages between the various educational segments leads to redundancy or gaps in the informational offerings. In medical school, a moat remains between the basic and clinical years; in fact, course content is frequently decided by a curriculum committee, without preliminary communication with responsible faculty members — integration apparently being expected to occur automatically at the level of the learner.

Fourth is the failure to distinguish between information essential for all physicians and that necessary only for specialists. This shortcoming is, in part, an outgrowth of the emphasis on inpatient rather than ambulatory care — so that the student experience resembles a mini-residency rather than an exposure to the problems nonspecialists are most likely to encounter in that field. The goal at this level is not to produce or recruit specialists but to develop a level of competence that might reasonably be expected of anyone who possesses an M.D. degree.

Another problem is the excessive use of residents for the teaching of medical students. This occurrence is perhaps the natural outcome of a faculty stressed by increasing bureaucratic detail and clinical responsibility. Since resident teaching is generally more interesting and rewarding, student instruction suffers.

Sixth, although clinical rotations are usually more popular than basic science courses, the educational ore is frequently low grade. Clinical clerks often function as "gofers" to perform the house officer's chores, without being given a meaningful role in patient care — although the balance between greater student responsibility and patient safety is delicate indeed.

Finally, there is insufficient exposure to ethics, economics, empathy, prevention, geriatrics, biostatistics, and medicolegal problems.

After graduation, the period of basic surgical or medical education suffers from many of the same difficulties that exist during the clinical years of medical school: short rotations are the rule, career interests often lie elsewhere, and specific curricular guidelines are missing. As a result of the lack of any explicit focus, the intern exists in educational purgatory between the students and the residents.

After one or more years of basic education, the final common pathway is entered. While graduate medical education satisfies many of the principles of adult learning, new difficulties arise.

The absence of a defined curriculum leads to an educational experience determined by certifying examinations, special interests of the faculty, and local patient populations.

A further problem is the programmatic rigidity produced by lockstep rotations, which makes it difficult to accommodate individual abilities, backgrounds, and goals. This inflexibility is particularly notable in large programs with many affiliated hospitals.

Of particular concern is the increasing emphasis on technical rather than scientific aspects of instruction, which tilts the educational balance toward action rather than understanding. Preoccupation with technique is an especial hazard for surgeons, since time spent in the operating room reduces time for other patient contacts that are equally important in the determination of surgical outcomes. As the sphere of activity of a surgeon shrinks to the operating room, he recedes from the realms of science and patient interaction.

Fellowship training, an extension of the residency period, has been allowed to grow like Topsy, with little coordination, control, supervision, or approval. Educational goals and objectives are poorly defined. Technology is overemphasized, and integration with parent disciplines is limited. Nevertheless, largely because it increases the technological depth of medical care, specialization is here to stay. The decision is not whether to have it, but how much can we afford?

The problems of content omission and/or

overlap in the educational continuum have been addressed by the development of curricular goals and objectives. The preparation of such objectives for each contact point reduces ambiguity, directs the educational experience for both the learner and the teacher, facilitates communication between those responsible for the various phases of the educational continuum, and guides evaluation, since testing can (and should) be based on such objectives.

Despite these advantages and strong support from educational theorists, learning objectives are not a panacea for the ills that beset teaching programs. The manner in which their content is presented is also critical. Because it emphasizes relevance and participation by the learner, a problem-solving mode is preferred. Teaching only by force-feeding facts into students like the proverbial Strasbourg goose produces a pâté that contains too much of the formulaic and too little of the spirit of science. In this regard, it should be remembered that the primary goal of teaching is to inspire students to want to know more; the secondary goal is to foster the development of critical and analytical abilities; and last is to impart information. The teacher who simply delivers facts is — since a student can read faster than a lecturer can talk — more of an impediment than an asset. Why do we persist? Because it is easier to impart information than to teach students how to think.

Largely because of time and curricular compression, topics such as ethics, medicine and the law, biostatistics, medical information systems, and medical economics are incompletely covered in medical school; but these subjects could be taught as a core curriculum for house officers. Shared educational experiences at the graduate level would enhance the quality and comprehensiveness of the instructional offerings in a time-effective manner.

We have not been as successful as we should have liked in integrating students and interns into patient care so that they, and we, feel that they are an essential part of the team with defined responsibilities. The art lies in enhancing this goal without sacrificing the quality of patient care.

At the graduate level, sufficient programmatic flexibility should exist to allow personalized educational experiences for each resident. There is a thin line between flexibility and chaos, but one can adjust for diverse background, goals, and abilities by fine-tuning individual learning opportunities if the program is not too large or broadly based.

The crowding out of science and other aspects of patient care by preoccupation with procedures may be avoided to a degree by greater use of trained technicians, which frees students and house officers for attendance at rounds, conferences, and seminars.

A final, and crucial, point is that the atmosphere in which curricular operations occur is much more important in fashioning the end product than the curriculum itself. It is critical to establish an environment in which scholarship is valued and rigorous intellectual discipline applied in both the investigative and clinical arenas. This emphasis should be apparent in conferences, on the wards, and in the operating room, as well as in the laboratory. It finds particular application in the journal club, which should be approached in a framework which emphasizes critical analysis rather than as a series of summaries of clinical content.

To produce physicians who blend the scientific method with appropriate values and skills, an informed and disciplined intellect is necessary. Humanitarianism is important, but compassion cannot atone for incompetence — nor need truth and knowledge exclude warmth. A poor physician is more often the product of error and sloppy thought than the failure to empathize. Only if he understands concepts and the process of rigorous analysis will the student be able to separate legitimate from unfounded conclusions. It is this approach to learning that we should be inculcating, rather than trying to deliver all of the information needed for a lifetime of practice.

Psychomotor Education
Point and Counterpoint

There can be little argument with the point that much of what is highest and best in medicine today has resulted from advances in technology. One need only consider the diagnostic power of magnetic resonance imaging and the therapeutic impact of surgical miniaturization to realize the claim of technology on medical care. Nor is this debt limited to the direct management of disease. Through

---

This article was published in a slightly different text in *The Journal of Bone and Joint Surgery*, 75-A:1263-1264, 1993.

---

technological adaptation, the computer has created the science of information management, which has become an adjunct indispensable to health care. Soon students will be growing up with high definition television and interactive programming. Having journals and textbooks accessible from the television screen, the classroom may shift to the home, spawning a new type of faculty career: the professorial media star. And we have not even considered the impact of virtual reality.

Given this level of wiring, it should not be surprising that technology — and its associated financial rewards — have tilted surgical education toward the "how's" rather than the "why's," toward *technique* rather than *understanding*. More time in the operating room has, however, reduced pre- and postoperative patient contact, which is also critical to surgical results. A patient's understanding, expectations, and needs must be explored and clarified prior to operative intervention; and extended guidance after surgery is often necessary for an optimal outcome.

The formal teaching of motor skills was initiated by Lippert and Murray, whose whip and chair efforts not only tamed the curricular tiger but also established the utility of motor skills laboratories for the education of orthopaedic surgeons.[1] However, as they noted, successful surgery entails more than manual competence. It is crucial to realize that precise and complete separation of motor skills from thought and subjective response is neither possible nor desirable. Hands are the servants of heart and head. In addition to coordinated and efficient movement, a surgeon should possess equanimity, confidence, perseverance, flexibility, and the capacity for honest self-appraisal — all tempered by a basic reluctance to operate. Essential cognitive attributes include knowledge of disease and patient, operative and nonoperative alternatives, the capacity for logical thought, and the ability to anticipate.

Knowledge of the effectiveness of a procedure is of particular import. As noted by a former mentor, if there is no indication for an operation, there is no indication for doing it well. The collision between proliferating health care technology and cost containment has stimulated intense public and legislative scrutiny of procedural interventions; as a result, limitations of cost will emphasize applications based on sound outcome studies, with a reduction in the number of operative interventions for the treatment of *effects* rather than causes. The employment of arthroscopy, for example, for shaving the retropatellar surface, will be challenged if long-term cost-effectiveness is not documented. And it is just possible that in seeking such documentation, we will find that shaving is more appropriate for the face than the patella, where, as befits cosmetic operations, its benefits may be more readily perceived.

Almost all treatments benefit *symptoms*; but only through double-blinded, randomized studies will we know which treatments affect the course of a disease. Achilles tenotomy may relieve claudication but could hardly be considered appropriate treatment for ischemic disease. Neither unaudited experience nor logical thought can replace controlled clinical trials, so until documentation of a procedure's effectiveness can be demonstrated, it should be considered a false idol and worship withheld. Unfortunately, American education is still heavily influenced by the stimulus-response model of Thorndike and Skinner: if a new instrument or procedure is offered, it is adopted; but surgeons are not rats or pigeons and should use their full intellectual abilities, avoiding seduction by anecdotal reports from "authorities" whose numerators are still in search of a denominator.

In addition to honing manual skills, psychomotor education should cultivate an understanding that new is not *better* until it is proven to be so. The medical roadside is littered with technologies that not only failed to improve but harmed patients; indeed, the initial enthusiasms for bloodletting, frontal lobotomy, and gastric freezing should give us pause to consider which of our current procedures will lie with these relics as the follies of our time.

While there is no single correct answer to the fundamental question of how much time should be purchased from other educational domains to teach manual skills, preoccupation with technique should not replace the time spent listening to, looking at, or touching the patient. To the extent that we permit the operative aspects of surgical education to diminish other essential clinical skills, to that extent will the humanistic base of surgical practice be eroded.

In spite of the growing tendency to equate surgery with procedural intervention, we must remember that surgery is more than the sum of its operations, however spectacular or ingenious; that neither the existence of an instrument nor the ability to perform an operation, however skillfully, is an indication for its employment; that technological prowess can help begin life, delay death, cure cancer, and repair or replace critical parts, but unless it is integrated harmoniously with the heart and head of a physician, modern medicine will fail to maintain a humanitarian counterpoint to the anvil chorus of technology.

References

1. Lippert, Frederick G. *Psychomotor Skills in Orthopaedic Surgery*. Baltimore: Williams & Wilkins, 1983.

In Search of the Tubercle Bacillus
The Death of Thomas Wolfe

Thomas Wolfe, who liked to have his fortune told, often asked Mrs. Jewett, who was very good at reading cards, to tell his fortune. He would stand behind her as she was dealing the cards, begin to wring his hands with nervousness, and then to pace up and down the room. "Mrs. Jewitt, if you see death there, don't tell me." Then he would come back and look over at the cards, "Is death there? Don't tell me if you see it." It was always on his mind, an early death. He

This essay was originally published in a slightly different text in *Mosaic* 20(3): 57–63, 1987.

thought he could never write down all he wanted to say.

Lamentably, foreboding became fact, although the cause of Wolfe's premature death has never been established. The theory that he died of tuberculosis of the brain, metastatic from a reactivated infection in his lungs, was challenged in 1974 by James Meehan who expressed the view that the seed of Wolfe's destruction had blossomed in the desert — that a dust-borne fungus called *Coccidioides immitis*, acquired during his tour of the Southwest, had struck Wolfe down. While this theory has the appeal of poetic prophecy, the medical premises upon which it is based are sufficiently questionable to justify further consideration.

Another reason for casting a medical eye on the events surrounding Wolfe's death was provided by the recent discovery, in the Wisdom Collection at Harvard, of the long-absent records from his hospitalization at Johns Hopkins between September 10, 1938, and his death five days later.

It is critical to understand that for the diagnosis of an infectious disease to be *definitive* the specific infectious agent must be recovered from the patient. If a microscopically specific expression of the organism is found on slides of the infected tissues, the diagnosis may be said to be *probable*. Less specific evidence, such as clinical or laboratory findings, allows only a *presumptive* diagnosis.

Thus, proof of the hypothesis that Wolfe died of a specific infectious disease would require recovery from Wolfe of the organism that caused that disease. There are two ways in which an organism may be retrieved from a patient: by culture or by finding it in smears prepared from diseased tissues. For reasons that are unclear, there are no culture reports in Wolfe's hospital records; nor were any organisms — bacterial or fungal — found in Wolfe's sputum or spinal fluid. One must realize, however, that these organisms are often difficult or impossible to find in such preparations, so the absence of proof does not constitute proof of absence.

Probable evidence for the diagnosis is also lacking: no unique pathologic reaction was found on the slides from Wolfe's brain. Both tuberculosis and coccidioidomycosis produce pathologic lesions known as granulomas or tubercles, although the tubercles of fungal infections usually bear more resemblance to an abscess than they do to tuberculosis. The pathologists at Johns Hopkins reported that several areas on the slides suggested early tubercle formation, but fully developed tubercles were not found. They, and the pathologists at the University of North Carolina who reviewed them more recently, concluded only that a meningitis was present, which might have been produced by any number of infectious agents, including bacteria (such as tuberculosis) or fungi (such as coccidioidomycosis).

We are thus left with presumptive evidence, which can be examined under the headings of probability, clinical, laboratory and x-ray manifestations, and findings at surgery.

With respect to probability, one must consider the likelihood that Wolfe developed tuberculosis as a result of living in Asheville for fifteen years, as opposed to the possibility that he acquired coccidioidomycosis from several days spent in the deserts of the Southwest. Asheville in 1900 had already become a world center for the treatment of tuberculosis. Known then as "The White Plague," tuberculosis was the most dreaded disease in the world and the leading cause of death in the United States. In 1920, Sir William Osler estimated that one-eighth of all deaths worldwide were due to this "Captain of the Men of Death" — and the "seed" was everywhere. It was estimated, for example, that one patient with advanced tuberculosis shed one to four billion organisms every twenty-four hours. With the seed so prevalent, the "soil" became the determinant of whether the bacteria flourished. Actually, the human body does not constitute a very favorable site for growth of the tubercle bacillus in the absence of such predisposing factors as nervous or physical exhaustion, debilitation, alcoholism, or chronic disease. The bacterium of tuberculosis is what is known as an obligate aerobe — meaning that it requires oxygen to flourish. Hence, the rarefied air of mountainous locations reduced the ability of the organism to survive and multiply and constituted the basis for climatotherapy, the only treatment available at that time. With the climate proclaimed as "tonic, invigorating, and bracing," thousands of tuberculosis victims flocked to Asheville — including George

Vanderbilt and E. W. Grove, who later contributed to the building of the city with the Biltmore House and the Grove Park Inn. The arrival of the railroad in 1880 contributed greatly to Asheville's accessibility, and brought, as well as patients, some twenty-five tuberculosis specialists — many of whom themselves had the disease. This influx of patients and physicians established Asheville as the foremost tuberculosis center in America.

Although the first tuberculosis sanitarium had been built in Asheville in 1871, there was still only one, the Old Winyah, when Thomas Wolfe was born in 1900. Between then and 1930, the number grew to twenty-five, providing over nine hundred beds; but most patients with tuberculosis stayed in boarding houses, where rates of fifteen dollars a week were only a third of those at the sanitaria. Such was the demand that the number of boarding houses rose from fifty-five in

1900 to a hundred and thirty-seven in 1910. Almost all of these establishments contained an open-air sleeping porch, which was a necessary advertising feature. Beginning in the 1930s, however, elimination of infected dairy cattle by the pasteurization of milk, improvement in living conditions and the development of antibiotics led to a gradual decline in the incidence of tuberculosis. Consequently, the sanitaria and most of the boarding houses slowly closed; by 1960 the tuberculosis era had ended.

The explosive need for boarding house facilities in Asheville following the turn of the century was not lost on Thomas Wolfe's mother, Julia, whose emergence as a woman of property began with her purchase of "My Old Kentucky Home" ("Dixieland" in *Look Homeward, Angel*) on August 30, 1906. She moved into the house promptly; but her husband, W. O., not a man of property, did not move with her — preferring the home he had built with his own hands two blocks away on Woodfin Street. His objections to the move were recorded in *Look Homeward, Angel*:

> It's a curse and a care, and the tax collector gets all you have in the end.

W. O. reviled and abused Eliza/Julia for her departure:

> You have deserted me in my old age; you have left me to die alone. Ah, Lord! It was a bitter day for us all when your gloating eyes first fell upon this damnable, this awful, this murderous and bloody Barn.

Eugene/Tom, being only six, was unable to shuttle as freely between the two houses as the other children, although he preferred the literal and figurative warmth of his father's home. His reaction to "that G-g-g-god-dam cold Barn" is recorded graphically in *Look Homeward, Angel*:

> The chilled white walls festered with damp: they drank in death from the atmosphere . . .
>
> Upstairs upon a sleeping porch, a thin-faced Jew coughed through the interminable dark . . .
>
> "In heaven's name, mama," Helen fumed, "Why do you take them in? Can't you see he's got the bugs?" "Why, no-o," said Eliza, pursing her lips. "He said he only had a little bronchial trouble."

Other passages in *Look Homeward, Angel* suggest that many of the visitors to My Old Kentucky Home had tuberculosis: one reference cites "the spot in the hall where the consumptive had collapsed in a hemorrhage." Another visitor was a man who "coughed gently behind his white hand . . . The boy did small services for him: he gave him a coin from week to week. He was a clothier from a New Jersey town. In the Spring, he went to a sanitarium; he died there later." Still later, Wolfe refers to a couple living in Dixieland:

> . . . a dissipated and alcoholic young man and a darkly handsome young woman, slightly tubercular."

Thus, it is highly unlikely that Thomas Wolfe, who lived for ten years in such a boarding house, could have escaped inhaling or ingesting the tubercle bacillus repeatedly while he was growing up. Once in the body, the bacterium is most likely to obtain a foothold in organs possessing a high concentration of oxygen, such as the lungs or brain. In the lungs, when defender cells, called macrophages, engulf and destroy the bacteria as rapidly as they are produced, the focus of infection usually becomes walled off, which reduces the supply of oxygen available to the bacteria and thereby halts their replication. In such a state of suspended activity, the organisms may exist for many years — like a weevil in a biscuit. However, the wall isolating this primary focus may be broken down at any time by other pathologic processes in the lung, such as pneumonia, whereby the tubercle bacilli escape into the bloodstream and lodge in other organs. In most of these organs, there is a tendency toward healing and regression. However, the infection is more difficult to control in the brain, and it usually spreads to the brain's coverings, or meninges, where it was, in Wolfe's day, invariably fatal. Tubercles developing on the meninges are often visible to the naked eye as grayish flecks, although in rapidly progressing infections, the full-blown pathologic picture may not have time to develop, which might account for the absence of classical microscopic findings in Wolfe's brain tissues.

Compared to the certainty that an Asheville

resident at the beginning of the twentieth century would have acquired a primary tuberculous infection, only about 50 percent of those who have lived for more than six months in the Southwest, where coccidioidomycosis is endemic, show evidence of a primary infection with this fungus. Since Wolfe lived in Asheville for fifteen years but traveled through the Southwestern deserts for only three or four days, the probability that he contracted coccidioidomycosis is considerably less than the likelihood that he developed a primary tuberculous infection. Furthermore, among men with primary coccidioidomycosis, only about one of every thousand died of it. Thus, from the standpoint of probability alone, the chances of Wolfe having succumbed to tuberculosis are greater by several orders of magnitude.

With respect to clinical findings, the initial symptoms of tuberculosis are often interpreted as a bad cold or the flu; however, a productive, occasionally blood-tinged, cough persists, while other symptoms — fever, night sweats, weight loss, and headaches — abate somewhat, leading to a false sense of recovery. The fever pattern characteristically has a broad daily swing, often fluctuating between 100 and 103 degrees. In its most virulent form, known colloquially as "galloping consumption," the attack begins suddenly with a chill, often just after exposure to cold or other debilitating circumstances. The temperature elevation is dramatic, and symptoms persist until death, which may occur in a matter of days or weeks. This latter clinical picture is quite similar to that manifested by Wolfe, whose final illness began with chills and a temperature of 105 degrees. Moreover, with meningeal involvement, convulsions, especially on one side, are common, as is paralysis of the ocular muscles, swelling of the optic nerves (the so-called choked disc) and various ab-normal reflexes — all of which Wolfe had during his illness.

Coccidioidomycosis is normally a benign and self-limited infection. Most patients never have symptoms. Those who do usually have a clinical picture similar to that of influenza. A prominent symptom is often joint pain, or arthralgia, which was not cited as one of Wolfe's complaints. Among patients in whom the disease progresses to the fatal, dissemi-nated form, ulcerating skin lesions are common; again, no such lesions were reported in Wolfe's records.

Another major clinical difference between tuberculosis and coccidioidomycosis lies in the course of the disease. Disseminated tuber-culosis with meningitis runs a fulminant course with death usually in a matter of weeks; how-ever, even in its fatal form, coccidioidal meningitis is characteristically much more subtle, with survival often for as long as two years. Wolfe's illness ran its course in ten weeks, during which time he was extremely sick. Thus, both the intensity and duration of his illness were more typical of tuberculosis.

There were in 1938 no laboratory tests that reliably distinguished tuberculosis from coccidioidomycosis; however, several non-specific changes in the blood and urine are more commonly found in one than the other. Wolfe had one early blood count that contained an elevation of a cell type (eosinophiles) more often seen in coccidioidomycosis; but a similarly non-specific urinary finding common in tuberculosis (albuminuria) also was found, so neither diagnosis was particularly favored by the laboratory studies.

Nor were the findings in x-rays of the lungs distinctive. Wolfe's chest x-rays showed a slowly shrinking pneumonic process in the upper portion of the right lung that never fully cleared.

Although most reactivated tuberculous lesions are found in the upper part of the lung, neither this finding, nor the generalized mottling observed in both lung fields, has precise diagnostic value.

Findings in the spinal fluid were more characteristic; in tuberculous meningitis, the number of cells in the spinal fluid ranges from 25 to 1,000, with over 50 percent of these cells being of a particular mononuclear variety. Wolfe's spinal fluid contained 230 cells, 75 percent of which were mononuclears. With fungal infections, the cell count is commonly higher, with more variation in cell type. Wolfe's surgeon, Dr. Walter Dandy, felt that the cell count in the spinal fluid alone was enough to make the diagnosis of tuberculosis.

Dr. Dandy's operative reports are very critical pieces of evidence. He described "myriads of tubercles" in the cerebellum, which he clearly ascribed to tuberculosis. As one of America's most eminent neurosurgeons, Dandy had seen tuberculosis of the brain often, so great credence must be given to his impressions at surgery. Since the way in which the tissue sections are prepared for study may affect the findings, it is possible that classical tubercles, even if present, would not be seen in the microscopic sections available for study. The validity of Dandy's surgical observations is enhanced by the knowledge that his preoperative diagnosis favored a brain abscess or a tumor that had metastasized to the brain. Tuberculosis, he thought, was less probable. Since he was looking primarily for evidence of other conditions, the sureness of his diagnosis of tuberculosis must be even more heavily weighed.

Thus, from the presumptive evidence available, the medical basis for the coccidioidomycosis theory must be questioned. The points cited by Meehan in support of this theory can be refuted as follows:

> It is "almost unknown" for someone who had tuberculosis of the lungs as a child to develop TB meningitis many years later.

Tuberculous meningitis can and does develop at any time after the initial infection, and the risk of its doing so is increased by a subsequent inflammatory process in the lung, such as pneumonia.

> Miliary tuberculosis of the brain usually brings death more quickly than was evidenced in Wolfe's case. The writer was ill for ten weeks; tuberculosis usually comes to its climax in four to six weeks.

Since we do not know exactly when in Wolfe's illness the organisms actually became disseminated, and since fatal miliary tuberculosis may run a longer course, it cannot be said that Wolfe's terminal illness was too long to be compatible with the diagnosis of tuberculosis. If, in fact, the onset of his headaches may be assumed to reflect the time of spread to the brain, there were about five weeks between the onset of headaches and Wolfe's death. Even if the interval were longer than usual, it is safer to bet on an uncommon manifestation of a common disorder than a typical presentation of an uncommon one.

The blood stain tests that preceded the operation of September 12 show no evidence of tuberculosis.

Tubercle bacilli or fungi are only rarely found on stained specimens of blood.

As late as September 10, the Hopkins staff was still considering three different diagnoses: "pulmonary neoplasm with cerebral metastases," "acute pulmonary tuberculosis," and "unresolved pneumonia with cerebral metastases."

This differential diagnosis was made on the day of Wolfe's admission to Hopkins, and before the exploratory surgery that led Dr. Dandy to change his diagnosis to tuberculosis.

> [A medical specialist cited by Meehan observed that] "in the final operation, Dr. Dandy found tubercles in some sections but not in others."

Tubercles anywhere would constitute probable evidence of either tuberculosis or coccidioidomycosis, but they were not confirmed microscopically.

> The pressure on Wolfe's brain and the large amount of water it was found to contain were caused by coccidioidal meningitis, not tuberculosis.

Hydrocephalus is also frequent in tuberculous meningitis; and as tuberculosis is much more common than coccidioidomycosis, the likelihood that the hydrocephalus was caused by tuberculosis is also considerably greater.

The onset of Wolfe's illness one day after he was exposed to the flu was too soon.

Since the incubation period for influenza is between one and four days, Wolfe's symptoms might well have been the result of his exposure the day before. Also since tuberculosis is an infectious disease, Wolfe *could* have developed it primarily at that time, without a preliminary bout of influenza.

Certainly there is poetic appeal in the notion that Wolfe foretold the means of his own death at the outset of *Look Homeward, Angel* when he wrote: "The seed of our destruction will blossom in the desert. . . ." The true irony, however, is that Wolfe died a respiratory death. Like Ben and W. O. — whose deaths he had described so poignantly — he literally drowned in his own secretions. Yet unlike W. O., who did not find the creative life before the black fog closed about him, and unlike Ben, who never captured the music of the lost world, Wolfe did recall for us the great forgotten language, the lost faces, the stone, the leaf, and the door.

References

1. Anderson, W. A. D. *Pathology*. St. Louis: C. V. Mosby, 1948.
2. Harrison, T. R., et al. *Principles of Internal Medicine*, 5th ed., New York: McGraw-Hill, 1966.
3. Hoagland, Mrs. Clayton. "Thomas Wolfe: Biography in Sound, NBC Radio Broadcast." Report in *The Carolina Quarterly* 9(1):5–19, 1956.
4. Medical records of Thomas Wolfe from the Johns Hopkins Hospital, Baltimore, Maryland, September 10–15, 1938, Shelfmark bMS AM 1883.9 (127), by permission of Mr. Paul Gitlin and of the Houghton Library, Harvard University, Cambridge, Massachusetts.
5. Meehan, J. "Seed of Destruction: The Death of Thomas Wolfe." *South Atlantic Quarterly* 73:173–83, 1974.
6. Osler, W., and T. McCrae. *The Principles and Practice of Medicine*. 9th ed., rev. New York: Appleton, 1920.
7. Stephens, I. "Asheville: The Tuberculosis Era." *North Carolina Medical Journal* 46:455–63, 1985.
8. Wolfe, Thomas. *Look Homeward, Angel*. New York: Scribners, 1929.
9. Wyngaarden, J. B., and L. H. J. Smith, eds. *Cecil Textbook of Medicine*. 2 vols. Philadelphia: W.B. Saunders, 1982, vol. 2.

THE VALUE OF STANDARDS
TO AN EMBATTLED PROFESSION

M any of us, I think, do not have a complete understanding of the role of American medical boards among health care organizations. Certainly prior to serving on one myself, I did not. I knew, of course, that it generated an examination that served as one of the rites of passage to medical adulthood; and while acknowledging the cognitive growth that resulted from this experience, I had not given much thought to the importance of the credentialing process to the public. As

This essay was originally published in *The Journal of Bone and Joint Surgery*. 70-A(10) (1988):1439–40.

a member of the Board, however, I came to realize that self-developed and enforced standards of learning are one of the pillars upon which any profession must rest.

Since credentialing has as its primary purpose protection of the public, it is also plain that these standards must be set and implemented apart from the friendly persuasions of those to whom they apply. While we cannot and should not operate in a vacuum, the perception of autonomy is crucial to the credibility of the certification process. Being practitioners themselves, board directors can never escape the personal implications of certification; but to the degree that conflict between public and private interest is answered in favor of the public, to that degree the boards achieve nobility of purpose.

Because they *are* accepted as independent and impartial, the specialty boards are recognized as potent and steadying influences in the embattled world of organized medicine. Residing between the halls of academe and the groves of specialty practice, the boards belong to neither world. Their beauty and their power are allied to their separation from these groups. Board members are elected by boards and are not expected to reflect any cognate relationship to the organizations that propose them or to their subspecialty disciplines.

Also, the purposes of a board differ from those of academic groups or specialty societies. Academics promote progress in specialty medicine through education and research; their constituents are the learners. Specialty societies determine the dimensions of the specialty and address the concerns of their members. Thus, the faculties who lead, the specialty societies who make the laws, and the boards who judge, have been likened to the executive, legislative, and judicial branches of the government. In this context, organizations such as the American Medical Association, the Association of American Medical Colleges, and the American College of Surgeons function as lobbyists for their own constituencies. Each of these arms provides balances and checks to the privileges of the other. This separation of duties is critical, since no one body can credibly lead, legislate, and judge.

It is evident that passing an examination following a residency does not assure competence in perpetuity. Basic information must be retained (and used) and new knowledge assimilated to maintain a high standard of practice. Therefore, periodic reassessment is rational and necessary. The problem is not with the concept but with the method. The certification process emphasizes cognitive mastery — what a physician knows — for which an examination is appropriate. For recertification, the principal concern is performance — what a physician does — which, because it reflects attitudes and skills as well as erudition, is more complex and difficult to quantify. Performance may be likened to an iceberg: the small, visible top, like knowledge, may be clearly seen and reliably measured; however, the greater, submerged part, composed of those qualities of humanism and character which determine how one's knowledge is used, is dimly perceived and defies precise description. This is the major challenge facing all specialty boards: how to measure performance reliably. Direct methods, such as medical record audits, on-site observation, and peer review, are limited by the difficulty in setting objective measurement criteria. Indirect methods, such as practice-based examinations or electronic simulations, are more quantifiable but have not been proven to parallel actual performance.

Thus, the search goes on. We will never find a perfect method, but that should not prevent our quest for a better one. Credentialing is a powerful tool that must not become so politically or emotionally entangled that it fails to serve the best interests of our patients. If medicine abdicates its responsibility to impose standards upon itself, we may be sure that our place will be taken by very interested, but less knowledgeable or understanding, others.

It is important to recognize the contributions of the boards to medical education and patient care. Those who have participated in the board movement should take great pride in what has been accomplished. To build upon this record of achievement, we must rededicate ourselves to the requirement of reasonable standards as a professional obligation and to use of the best means possible to meet that responsibility.

MEDICINE IN THE THIRD MILLENIUM
WHAT THEN MUST WE DO?

I n ancient Rome, citizens celebrated the New Year by an exchange of coins. The coins contained the image of Janus, for whom January was named, and who, by his two-faced profile, was able to see forward and backward — the future as well as the past.

Our labors in the medical vineyards during the past hundred years have been remarkably productive, and although our ability to recognize, manage, and prevent medical disorders will undoubtedly continue to increase, there will be changes in the climate and in the vineyards themselves. Change, after all, is natural; it is fixity that is unnatural. So with past as preview, we might look at the century ahead to anticipate the effect of these environmental changes on medicine and its practice.

Some changes, such as physician-to-population and generalist-to-specialist ratios, are functional. They represent the ebb and flow of societal currents and rarely have permanent effects. These cyclical variations must be distinguished from structural changes, which are more deeply rooted and require decisive intervention for modification.

One of the most menacing structural alterations in medicine is that resulting from the insertion of third parties between physicians and their patients. The intrusion of insurance companies, lawyers, and bureaucrats has moved the dollar bill, once outside and after, to a place between and before the physician-patient encounter, thereby undermining the professional nature of the relationship. Pre-paid health plans, by contributing to patients' perception that they are receiving their health care from a corporation rather than an individual, will further erode the natural bond between physician and patient.

Limited resources are likely to have other structural effects upon medicine: a return to multiple levels of medical care; rationing of expensive technologies, and some form of nationalized health care. Being less costly, more medical service will be provided by generalists, and, in a reversal of the past, doctors will be criticized more often for under- than overtreatment. As a result of diminished autonomy and reduced economic prospects for physicians, the quality of applicants to medical school may fall — an event perhaps heralded by the lower grade-point averages and Medical College Admission Test scores of those applying in recent years.

Economic constraints will also be felt in research. Increasing competition for diminishing grant support will escalate the pressure to publish at the expense of sound and original work. Fraud in research is likely to become more frequent, as is the introduction of new procedures that have not been sufficiently tested to determine their indications and effectiveness of the socioeconomic implications of their use.

With the world's population expected to increase by over 20 percent in the next decade, the accompanying demand for medical resources will generate enormous economic pressure in the health care system. It would be reassuring to believe that physicians were the victims, rather than the agents, of this economic strain; however, by accenting personal concerns, physicians have contributed to the fiscal noose that encircles the neck of medicine. (I don't think I have to tell you who holds the other end of the rope.) The tension between entrepreneurship and altruism has always been a threat to the professional ethic of medicine; how this conflict between cost and care is resolved, whether we first serve self or public interest, will determine whether medicine retains its place of honor among the professions. Our personal values determine the level at which we employ our abilities and skills, and these values are tested every day. Should we certify the necessity for private-duty nursing? Ought we to extend a period of disability? Every time we use the word "should" or "ought," we imply an ethical issue. The answer to any single question may not alter the earth in its orbit, but the sum of these decisions will decide the plane upon which medicine is practiced.

In addition to the impact of economic forces, our medical consciences will be increasingly impacted by external value systems, changing societal perceptions, technological eruption, and decreasing educational breadth. The introduction of new value systems has made moral judgement more complex. In the past, *physicians* determined how medicine was practiced; now lawyers, bureaucrats, other health professionals, insurers, and patients have their own concept of medicine. As these interpretations multiply and diverge, the search for a unifying ethic becomes more critical and more difficult.

Physicians must also deal with conflict in their personal value systems. Consider the tension between the physician's roles as healer and as scientist. As healer, he is obligated to act in the best interest of the individual patient; as scientist, the physician must respect the precepts of valid experimentation, which may entail suboptimal treatment of individual patients to assure optimal therapy for all patients.

Changing societal perceptions have also created ethical controversies. The current notion that blame must be fixed for anything less than a perfect result has led to an unfair tort system and astronomical malpractice rates. While the distinction between unfortunate and unreasonable outcomes is often blurred, these judgements must be made, and clearly others, including patients themselves, must assume outcome responsibility. A person dies, after all, not just of his disease, but of his entire life.

Most solutions create their own set of problems, and technological answers to medical problems have been no exception. The eruption of procedural methodologies has created a bewildering panoply of choices that did not exist previously. Consider the ethical dilemmas posed by our increased capacity to extend life and our commitment to relieve suffering; or between our ability to enhance the quality of life and the need to conserve resources — especially when we learn that the frequency with which a technology is used is directly related to its reimbursement level.

The proliferation of technologies has also encouraged specialization, which, in turn, has lead to a loss of educational breadth. With knowledge in depth, one automatically purchases ignorance in breadth, resulting in less comprehension of the world around us and of the relatedness of the parts to the whole. Patients become disembodied appendages or specimens — at which moment they cease to be human beings. The vocationally-oriented training of specialization has immediate application — the quick fix. The liberal arts, lacking practical relevance, are not perceived as necessary. How can philosophy compete with the glamour of computer science? Greek and Latin, which always struggled to hold their own, have almost disappeared from the curriculum; in their place are words, and more words, which often seem to be a substitute for thought rather than a means of expressing it. Remembering that the Ten Commandments required only 297 words and the Gettysburg Address 266, one must wonder about a federal directive to regulate the price of cabbage that contains 26,911 words. Lacking exposure to the concision of Latin grammar, students fail to develop the logic and stylistic economy needed for clear expression. But we are better at numbers; so good, in fact, that a patient's status is often reported numerically, and therapy based on formulas that will produce "good numbers." The person is almost superfluous; even experienced practitioners treat patients on the basis of "objective data" rather than the "anecdotal testimony" of the patient himself.

What then must we do to preserve the ethical dimension that accounts for medicine's place of distinction as a profession — to resolve the deepening conflicts between personal and public interest, between our professional obligation to provide optimal care and economic constraints, between the best treatment and the patient's right to decide, or between the physician as healer and the physician as scientist? These are not issues that may be dealt with reflexly; they have varying dimensions that defy stereotypic answers. Whether or not these precepts can be taught, other than by example, is debatable; even if they can, not all of the answers are known. And certainly knowledge of ethical principles does not ensure their proper use.

These reservations notwithstanding, I should like to offer the following ethical ballast for the turbulent waters ahead:

First, the patient's welfare must be given highest priority. Self-interest must not be allowed to precede altruism or objectivity, even though powerful forces are driving today's physicians toward private rather than public concerns. If we become a broker for third parties rather than an advocate for patients, we will sacrifice the public trust so critical to the high position that medicine has held in the past. This is not to imply that we can ignore economic considerations in health care decisions. Medical resources, like the grass in a pasture, are limited. It may seem harmless enough to add a few private cows to the medical pasture, but if everyone acts in the same manner, the medical commons will soon be exhausted. Irresponsible individual action can thus decimate the entire medical community. By applying the principle of universality — that is, by stopping to consider the effect of a personal action becoming a universal mode of behavior — the inherent propriety of an act may be better understood.

We must also be aware of a second current that threatens the foundations of patient care: that of allowing the means of competition for patients to become institutional or personal ends for the creation of practice monopolies. The ends must remain access and quality of medical care.

Third, we must understand that it is perfectly acceptable for a patient to refuse a specific recommendation for therapy, even if this decision does not seem to be in his best interest, provided the patient has sufficient knowledge and awareness to make an informed decision. There is no reason for a terminally ill patient to be maintained indefinitely as a heart-lung preparation, which, like pasting summer's leaves on winter's trees, is unseemly as well as impractical.

For the surgeon, however, the obverse may be ethically more difficult and ultimately more dangerous. A surgeon's bias is toward surgery, so when a referring physician offers to admit, work up, and look after a surgical patient postoperatively, leaving only the operation for the surgeon, the tendency to concur is strong. The surgeon can do what he likes most, and for which he is best paid. The eventual damage to the profession is, however, hard to over-estimate. Surgery requires input from head and heart, as well as hands. If surgeons be-come simply motor end-organs for someone else's cerebral cortex, they will have compromised the future of surgery — and their own integrity — for a few dollars more.

Fourth, although specialization has swung the educational pendulum toward depth in learning, a horizontal dimension must be preserved to permit sound ethical judgements.

Specialization, at least to the organ sys-tem level, usually enhances medical care. It is philosophically less rational beyond that point, leading to a loss of intellectual wholeness. Seeking freedom from modulating influences is human nature, but the resulting isolation reduces cross-fertilization and fosters perception of the patient as a part rather than a person. Thus, continuing fragmentation of medicine, while improving therapy for a particular disorder may lead to an overall reduction in patient care. For physicians to enjoy the status of professionals, they must demonstrate their capacity to serve society's broad needs. If medical schools, driven by the centrifugal force of specialization, become divorced from the rest of the educational community, they will have turned back toward the proprietary schools of the pre-Flexnerian era. To prevent this professional separation, the baccalaureate curriculum must be more thoughtfully folded into the continuum of medical education. There is presently too little coordination between collegiate advisors and medical school admissions committees; too many courses are taken to improve grade-point averages or ease the passage to medical school, rather than to provide a base that will accommodate both the science and the art of medicine. By limiting the number of humanities majors accepted to medical school, we are spawning one-dimensional scientists who often cannot integrate their science into the world around them. To encourage premedical students to take non-scientific courses, earlier decisions should be made on their applications to medical school; they could then take such subjects with less concern about the grades they make. A general education allows us to enjoy life through a greater variety of cerebral inputs: music, literature, art, and drama, to mention a few. Further, students who understand the role and relationships of different disciplines are more likely to view ethical issues in the broad context they require. They will be able to recognize and discard superficial answers, and they will understand that they cannot overlook evidence that refutes their biases. They will better appreciate that a fact exists only in the context of a person, and the skill of a physician relates to his ability to give that fact appropriate dimension and location within a human being.

The peril of means becoming ends also exists in the educational arena. As we have acquired powerful teaching tools, there has been a shift toward emphasis on process rather than purpose of education; but, however elegant, videotapes and self-instructional programs cannot replace the inspiration and individualization afforded by personal interaction between teacher and learner.

Last, we must recognize that reliable epidemiological data must be available before treatments are adopted for widespread use. It may be argued that failure to employ intuitively or anecdotally efficacious therapy denies or delays optimal care, but without randomized clinical trials, we do not know what optimal care is. While thoroughly informed consent and the patient's right to decide must be respected, carefully designed and monitored human studies are critical for the progress of clinical medicine. Unwarranted assumptions are rampant, even upon the printed page. Authors and editors have a moral responsibility to address the questions of validity, generalizability, and economic practicality when new therapies are presented. The medical roadside is littered with abandoned therapies whose initial use was suggested by judgement or logic: remember gastric freezing for peptic ulcers, ligation of the internal mammary artery for coronary artery disease, the "button operation" for ascites, and frontal lobotomies — or, closer to home, Boplant and Ostamer. After wide dissemination, such procedures are not easily withdrawn — even by an author with the integrity to debunk his own inventions. By testing the efficacy of new treatments, science can be lifted from the fog of empiricism. Such studies will not guarantee an optimal outcome, but, since clinical epidemiology is based in probability, they are more likely to lead to success.

In conclusion, I urge you to resist separation from your patients by economic concerns, to examine personal action in the light of universal application, to maintain the dimension of breadth in your continuing education, and to insist upon valid outcome studies before employing new technologies. Noble purposes are fragile and easily overcome by materialistic concerns; in the end, however, it is the placement of giving in front of taking that will make the difference. If we follow this principle, the quality of medical care will not only endure in the third millennium, it will prevail.